# Table of Contents

# Introduction

The terms used for the bipolar extremes, 'melancholy' (depression) and 'mania' both have their origins in Ancient Greek. 'Melancholy' derives from melas 'black' and chole 'bile', because Hippocrates thought that depression resulted from an excess of black bile. 'Mania' is related to menos 'spirit, force, passion'; mainesthai 'to rage, go mad'; and mantis 'seer', and ultimately derives from the Indo-European root men- 'mind' to which, interestingly, 'man' is also sometimes connected. ('Depression', the clinical term for melancholy, is much more recent in origin and derives from the Latin deprimere 'press down' or 'sink down'.)

The idea of a relationship between melancholy and mania can be traced back to the Ancient Greeks, and particularly to Aretaeus of Cappadocia, who was a physician and philosopher in the time of Nero or Vespasian (first century AD). Aretaeus described a group of patients that who 'laugh, play, dance night and day, and sometimes go openly to the market crowned, as if victors in some contest of skill' only to be 'torpid, dull, and sorrowful' at other times. Although he suggested that both patterns of behaviour resulted from one and the same disorder, this idea did not gain currency until the modern era.

The modern psychiatric concept of bipolar disorder has its origins in the nineteenth century. In 1854, Jules Baillarger (1809–1890) and Jean-Pierre Falret (1794–1870) independently presented descriptions of the disorder to the Académie de Médicine in Paris. Baillarger called the illness folie à double forme ('dual-form insanity') whereas Falret called it folie circulaire ('circular insanity'). Falret observed that the disorder clustered in families, and correctly postulated that it had a strong genetic basis.

In the early 1900s the eminent German psychiatrist Emil Kraepelin (1856–1926) studied the natural course of the untreated disorder and found it to be punctuated by relatively symptom-free intervals. On this basis he distinguished the disorder from démence précoce (schizophrenia) and coined the term 'manic–depressive psychosis' to describe it. Kraepelin emphasized that, in contrast to démence précoce, manic–depressive psychosis had an episodic course and a more benign outcome.

Interestingly, Kraepelin did not distinguish between people with both manic and depressive episodes and people with only depressive episodes with psychotic symptoms. This distinction dates back only to the 1960s, and is largely responsible for the modern emphasis on bipolarity, and hence on mood elevation, as the defining feature of the disorder.

The terms 'manic–depressive illness' and 'bipolar disorder' are comparatively recent, and date back from the 1950s and 1980s respectively. The term 'bipolar disorder' (or 'bipolar affective disorder') is thought to be less stigmatizing than the older term 'manic–depressive illness', and so the former has largely superseded the latter. However, some psychiatrists and some people with bipolar disorder still prefer the term 'manic–depressive illness' because they feel that it reflects the nature of the disorder more accurately.

## WHAT IS BIPOLAR?

Bipolar disorder is a mental health disorder that can cause dramatic changes in mood and energy levels. Symptoms can affect daily life severely. Spotting the signs of bipolar disorder can help a person to get treatment.

The person's mood can range from feelings of elation and high energy to depression. There can also be disruption in sleep and thinking patterns and other behavioral symptoms.

The extremes of mood are known as manic episodes and depressive episodes.

Hypomania has symptoms of a manic episode that are less severe.

According to the National Alliance on Mental Illness (NAMI), people receive a diagnosis on average at the age of 25 years, but symptoms can appear during the teenage years, and less commonly, during childhood.

This is a form of mental health disease where a person faces extreme kinds of mood swings. This comprises of both high, manic periods and low, depressive episodes. It is also referred to as manic depression where the mood swings are not only unpredictable but also extreme. From affecting a person's work-life to ruining relationships, the severity of this problem is huge. Three different types of symptoms can be faced with bipolar disorder including depression or alcoholism, hypomania, and mania. Sometimes bipolar disorder patients display an array of psychosis-related symptoms. This includes hallucinations (hearing or seeing things which aren't even there) and delusions (false fixed beliefs in things which aren't true). The highs and lows that bipolar disorder brings with are massive.

Signs and symptoms

Symptoms of mania include euphoria.

Bipolar disorder is a condition with mood swings that can range from euphoria to depression.

However, for a diagnosis of bipolar I disorder, a person only needs to have a manic episode.

In fact, a person with bipolar I disorder may never experience a major depressive disorder, despite the name bipolar.

Signs of mania

When someone has mania, they do not just feel very happy. They feel euphoric.

A person with mania may:

• have a lot of energy

• feel able to do and achieve anything

• have difficulty sleeping

• use rapid speech that jumps between topics and ideas

• feel agitated, jumpy, or "wired"

- engage in risky behaviors, such as reckless sex, spending a lot of money, dangerous driving, or unwise consumption of alcohol and other substances

- believe that they are more important than others or have important connections

- show anger or aggression if others challenge their views or behavior

Severe mania can involve psychosis, with hallucinations or delusions. Hallucinations can cause a person to see, hear, or feel things that are not there.

People may have delusions and distorted thinking that cause them to believe that certain things are true when they are not.

They may believe, for example, that they have important friends (such as the president of the United States) or that they descend from royalty.

A person in a manic state may not realize that their behavior is unusual, but others may notice a change in behavior. Some may see the person's outlook as sociable and fun-loving, while others may find it unusual or bizarre.

The individual may not realize that they are acting inappropriately or be aware of the potential consequences of their behavior.

They may need help in getting help and staying safe.

## Hypomania

Not everyone will have a severe manic episode. Less severe mania is known as hypomania. Symptoms are similar to those of mania, but the behaviors are less extreme, and people can often function well in their daily life.

If a person does not address the signs of hypomania, it can progress into a more severe form of the condition at a later time.

## Depression

During a low phase, a person may feel depressed and unable to do anything.

Signs of a depressive episode are the same as the symptoms of a major depressive episode.

They may include:

- feeling down or sad

- having very little energy

- having trouble sleeping or sleeping a lot more than usual

- thinking of death or suicide

- forgetting things

- feeling tired

- losing enjoyment in daily activities

- having a "flatness" of emotion that may show in the person's facial expression

In severe cases, a person may experience psychosis or a catatonic depression, in which they are unable to move, talk, or take any action.

Although rare, bipolar disorder could occur in young children and teenagers.

In children

Bipolar disorder is a lifelong condition. It can be present in young children, although it often does not emerge later, often in the late teens or early adulthood.

This may happen when a trigger causes clear signs of mania or depression, but often there is no clear trigger.

It can be hard to detect bipolar disorder in toddlers or young children, as children of this age often display uncontrolled behavior until they learn new ways of behaving. This has led to controversy over the diagnosis of bipolar disorder in young children.

Children with bipolar disorder may have severe temper tantrums that can last for hours, possibly with signs of aggression. These may not improve with age, as bipolar disorder makes it harder than others to learn alternative behaviors.

Parents may also notice periods of extreme happiness and silly moods in their child.

At this age, the signs of bipolar disorder may resemble those of another condition, such as attention deficit hyperactivity disorder (ADHD).

Teens

Teenagers may show some of the more common signs of bipolar disorder, especially an increase in risky behaviors, such as:

- reckless sexual activity, drug or alcohol use

- poor performance in school

- fighting

- thinking more about death or suicide

It is important that any young person showing these symptoms sees a mental health professional.

Learn more here about how bipolar disorder can affect teens.

Causes

Doctors do not know exactly what causes bipolar disorder, but the following appear to play a role:

Genetic factors: A person with bipolar disorder may have a parent with the condition. However, having a parent or even a twin with bipolar disorder does not mean a person will have it.

Stress: Someone who has a genetic predisposition may experience their first episode of depression or mania during or after a time of severe stress, for example, the loss of a job or a loved one.

Should I see a doctor?

It is always a good idea to speak with a doctor when there is concern about severe mood swings that seem to come and go or make it difficult to work.

The best person to start with may be a primary care physician or family doctor. However, they will likely refer someone with these symptoms to a psychiatrist, or a specialist who cares for people with mental health disorders.

Someone who notices these symptoms in a friend or loved one can also speak with their doctor about their concerns. The doctor can help find local support groups or other mental health resources.

Suicide risk

Risk-taking and thinking about suicide can pose real dangers for a person with bipolar disorder.

Whenever there is a possibility of harm or suicide, it is important to address the concern quickly and directly.

If there is an imminent risk, someone should contact the local police or suicide crisis hotline immediately.

Suicide prevention

- If you know someone at immediate risk of self-harm, suicide, or hurting another person:

- Call 911 or the local emergency number.

- Stay with the person until professional help arrives.

- Remove any weapons, medications, or other potentially harmful objects.

- Listen to the person without judgment.

- If you or someone you know is having thoughts of suicide, a prevention hotline can help. The National Suicide Prevention Lifeline is available 24 hours a day at 1-800-273-8255.

## Related conditions

Bipolar disorder has a number of comorbidities, or conditions that often occur alongside it.

Other mental health conditions that people might experience include:

• anxiety

• posttraumatic stress disorder (PTSD)

• ADHD

• misuse of alcohol and other substances

These can complicate the diagnosis.

It can take time to receive a correct diagnosis of bipolar disorder, as a doctor may identify one of these conditions, or a personality disorder, instead.

If the person experiences psychosis, this can sometimes lead to a misdiagnosis of schizophrenia, a mental health disorder marked by persistent hallucinations and delusions.

Treating these conditions may make it more difficult to diagnose or treat bipolar disorder. It can also take time to find a suitable medication and the correct dose for the individual.

However, once a person receives a correct diagnosis and appropriate treatment, medication can help to control the symptoms of bipolar disorder, and these related conditions usually improve as well.

Types of bipolar disorder

The Diagnostic and Statistical Manual of Mental Disorders Fifth Edition (DSM-5) describes four types of bipolar disorder.

1. Bipolar I disorder

This involves periods of mania that last at least 7 days, or any duration if the person is hospitalized.

If a person experiences severe manic or depressive episodes, they may need emergency treatment in the hospital to prevent harm to themselves or to others, for example through reckless behavior.

2. Bipolar II disorder

A person with bipolar II disorder has episodes of depression and hypomania. Hypomania is less extreme than a full manic episode.

People with bipolar II disorder tend to not have full mania.

Learn more here about the differences between type I and II bipolar disorder.

### 3. Cyclothymic disorder

Someone with cyclothymic disorder will also have alternating periods of hypomania and depression lasting for at least 2 years.

The main difference between cyclothymic disorder and bipolar II is that the symptoms of a person with cyclothymia tend to be less severe and do not meet the criteria for hypomania and depression.

4. Other specified and unspecified bipolar disorders

A person may have bipolar disorder that does not fit within the above patterns. They may receive a diagnosis of either "other specified bipolar disorder" or "unspecified bipolar disorder," depending on their symptoms.

## Diagnosis

A doctor will talk to the person about their symptoms and use the DSM-5 criteria to make a diagnosis.

In order to diagnose bipolar disorder, a healthcare provider should begin with a complete medical interview and a physical exam to rule out a physical cause for the person's behaviors.

There is currently no blood test or imaging that can diagnose the condition, but a doctor may suggest tests to rule out other medical conditions that might have similar symptoms.

If no medical conditions or medicines are causing the symptoms, the healthcare provider will consider bipolar disorder. They may refer the person to a mental health specialist.

The best person to diagnose bipolar disorder is a psychiatrist or psychiatric nurse practitioner who specializes in the care of people with mental health disorders.

## Treatment

Prescribers usually treat bipolar disorder with a combination of medications and talk therapy, or psychotherapy.

Because bipolar disorder is a lifelong disease, treatment should also be lifelong.

Medications

Medications for treating bipolar disorder include:

• mood stabilizers, such as lithium and some antiseizure medicines

- antipsychotics, to help manage mania and psychotic symptoms

- antidepressants may be used in some cases, depending on the person's symptoms and other considerations

It can take time to find a suitable medication and dose for the individual.

Some people discontinue their medication because it has adverse effects. If adverse effects occur, it is essential to speak to the prescriber, who may be able to change the dose or treatment. Discontinuation of medications for bipolar disorder can result in a return of symptoms.

Some people discontinue the medication because they miss the "highs" that bipolar disorder brings. They may feel they are no longer "themselves." People with this condition may be highly creative during a manic or hypomanic phase, and they may miss this aspect of their personality.

People with bipolar disorder are more likely to approach a doctor with depression than with mania.

Some treatments for depression can trigger an initial manic phase in a person who has the condition. This first experience of mania may be the first sign that a person has bipolar disorder.

# Talking therapy

Counseling or cognitive behavioral therapy (CBT) can help a person with bipolar disorder, as it can make them more aware of the negative aspects of their behavior and of triggers that could sabotage their treatment, such as substance use.

Learning tips for getting enough sleep, dealing with stress, and establishing a steady work-life balance may all help to control mood changes.

Electroconvulsive therapy

If medication and talk therapy are not effective in managing the symptoms of bipolar disorder, a psychiatrist may consider electroconvulsive therapy (ECT).

In ECT, a doctor applies a controlled electric shock to certain areas of the brain in order to cause a seizure. Doctors do not know exactly how it works, but there is evidence that ECT can help to regulate mood and other symptoms.

A doctor will only recommend it if symptoms are severe, if medication and counseling do not work, or if the person is unable to take or tolerate medication.

## Living with bipolar disorder

Bipolar disorder is a lifelong disorder that can have a severe impact on the individual and their family and friends.

Getting help early and actively participating in treatment are the keys to successfully managing this condition.

Though therapy and prescription medications are often helpful, there is an entire grey area regarding the effectiveness of CBD on this problem. Does science prove CBD useful in treating such condition?

## CBD OIL FOR BIPOLAR DISORDER

Bipolar disorder can be described as a manic-depressive brain illness. This disorder causes unusual changes in energy levels and mood and it can cause serious disruption of the daily life of a person. Currently, the severe condition is considered genetic and it may be worsened or triggered by substance abuse. Antidepressants and anti-psychotic pharmaceuticals are used to relieve bipolar disorder. However, over half of bipolar patients don't believe in the full effectiveness of these medications. That's why many people are turning to natural remedies like CBD.

Studies have shown that CBD provides neuroprotection in chronic and acute neurodegenerative disorders. Currently, there are published studies that show that free radical generation and oxidative stress may have an important role to play in bipolar disorder pathogenesis. In-vivo, as well as in-vitro studies, have confirmed the neuroprotective properties of CBD.

RESEARCH RESULTS ON THE NEUROPROTECTIVE PROPERTIES OF CBD

CBD exerts neuroprotective and antioxidative benefits in human beings. CBD has therefore been found to inhibit oxidative damage and increased brain-derived neurotrophic (BDNF) factor levels. BDNF is important for synaptic plasticity and therefore neuro-protection. When CBD mitigates oxidative stress, it prevents or potentially relieves bipolar symptoms.

Today, there are many bipolar patients that have used CBD to relieve symptoms of this disorder or to reduce the adverse effects of the conventional therapeutic drugs for improving the symptoms of it. Basically, there is evidence that shows the effectiveness of CBD in improving the symptoms of bipolar disorder. Nevertheless, anti-drug campaigns and stringent laws make conducting properly controlled and large-scale studies difficult. This has limited the exploration of the anti-psychotic benefits of CBD and its effective use in improving the symptoms of bipolar disorder.

## REALITY OF USING CBD TO RELIEVE BIPOLAR DISORDER

Bipolar disorder is among the oldest illnesses that are known in this world with records dating back thousands of years.

However, modern doctors face a major challenge when trying to relieve this condition. Drug abuse is the major challenge to the therapeutic aid of bipolar disorder. And, this problem affects six percent of the entire population but it plagues over fifty percent of bipolar patients. Interestingly, CBD seems to be the most preferred drug for improving the symptoms of bipolar disorder. But, many people question the role of this cannabinoid in improving the symptoms of bipolar disorder.

Should you consider CBD as a form of treatment?

The most commonly used form of cannabis is CBD oil. This natural, plant-based extract comprises of phytochemicals referred to as cannabinoids. The cannabinoids are the feel-good molecules which are naturally produced by the body. It brings about a secure and relaxed feeling with it while we engage in an array of activities. From keeping our body well-oiled and functioning to reducing inflammation, ensuring the proper functioning of our intestines and stomach, and modulation of pain – it does unbelievable things. This is the reason why researchers wanted to take a good hard look at how CBD can improve bipolar disorder.

Bipolar Disorder and its several varieties are resistant to treatment which explains the rate of disability. Therefore,

CBD has been investigated to see whether it is of benefit in treating such disorder.

The postmortem studies conducted on the human brain shows that when patients are diagnosed with different types of mental illnesses including Bipolar Disorder, abnormalities in the endocannabinoid system are found.

## The role of CBD in Bipolar-associated psychosis

Scientists believe that the antipsychotic effects of CBD could be therapeutic in patients with bipolar-associated psychotic symptoms. Moreover, reports show that CBD has anticonvulsant properties and exhibits protective effects against glutamate toxicity and may have a mood-stabilizing action similar to some anticonvulsants of proven value in Bipolar Affective Disorder (BAD).

Recently, some authors suggested that CBD has potential antipsychotic effects. This was confirmed by the observation that CBD acted in a similar way to haloperidol in animal tests predictive of antipsychotic activity. Moreover, a placebo-controlled case study of one patient with schizophrenia (intolerant to haloperidol) revealed antipsychotic effects of high-dose oral CBD. The patient experienced 60% to 69% improvement in his symptoms within 4 weeks of CBD therapy.

The impact of CBD on Bipolar disorder's manic and hypomanic episodes

Unfortunately, the evidence regarding the use of CBD in bipolar disorder remains very limited. However, the effects of cannabis use on bipolar disorder symptoms have been investigated. More than 70% of people with bipolar affective disorder have reported trying cannabis, and around 30% of them use it regularly. Unsuccessfully, the authors of this study reported that the regular use of cannabis was associated with earlier onset of bipolar disorder. It also resulted in poorer outcomes and fluctuations in an individual's cycling patterns and severity of manic or hypomanic episodes.

More research is warranted in order to see whether supplementing CBD might help alleviate some of the negative effects of cannabis use. Also, additional research is needed to determine whether CBD on its own might provide some beneficial effects on people with bipolar affective disorder.

## The Connection Between Cannabis and Bipolar Disorder

Research into the relationship between cannabis and bipolar disorder has resulted in contradictory results: some studies say using cannabis improves cognitive functions, with patients reporting that it works better than conventional drugs to treat their mania and depression. But other studies suggest it increases depressive symptoms and that continued use of cannabis is associated with a higher occurrence of manic episodes. And there's the risk, too, of dependence and drug abuse—research has found that people with bipolar disorder are 6.8 times more likely to have a history of illicit marijuana use than the rest of the population.

Despite all this, the father from the United Patients Group may have been onto something. While case studies on cannabis' effects have been mixed, there's a lot of evidence that CBD has the same antipsychotic and anticonvulsive properties as conventional bipolar disorder treatments. In other words, the chemical makeup of the strain you use does seem to matter, especially the balance of cannabis' two most famous ingredients: tetrahydrocannabinol (THC) and cannabidiol (CBD).

## The Difference Between THC and CBD

Of the 113 known compounds in marijuana, THC and CBD are the two principal active cannabinoids. Both interact with the endocannabinoid system in your body, the system that affects mood, appetite, pain sensation, and memory (this system is also known to play a role in mental disorders when it doesn't function properly). The amount of THC and CBD in your cannabis—plus the way these compounds interact with each other—

results in the different "highs" you get from various strains.

So, how do these two compounds differ? It's a surprisingly long list. THC is psychoactive and has properties that relieve pain, reduce vomiting, and reduce muscle spasms. It also has a relaxing effect on most people, which can give you that classic "stoned" feeling. And while marijuana doesn't cause psychotic disorders (contrary to familiar old-school propaganda), research shows that it canmimic symptoms—and this effect also comes from THC.

CBD also relieves pain, and it has additional properties that are anti-anxiety, anti-inflammatory, and neuroprotective. But even more interesting are CBD's antipsychotic and anticonvulsive properties, which suggest the compound could be used to replace conventional antipsychotics and anticonvulsants, the two drug classes most commonly prescribed to people with bipolar disorder. For instance, CBD's antipsychotic properties mean that the cannabinoid acts like an "atypical" antipsychotic—working similarly to a conventional antipsychotic medication but without the same serious, long-term side effects.

So while THC can induce psychotic reactions and impair cognitive functions, CBD's antipsychotic properties mitigate the effects of THC. It makes sense, then, that a strain with a high CBD content would be effective against bipolar disorder, while a strain with high THC might only aggravate psychotic symptoms. But unless you specifically seek out a high-CBD marijuana, it's likely you'll wind up with a strain that's much higher in THC. In a study from the University of Mississippi that assessed the THC/CBD content of illegal marijuana confiscated between 1994 and 2014, researchers found that THC content increased from 4% to 12% over the years, while CBD decreased. There used to be about 14 times more THC than CBD in marijuana—now there's 80 times more.

## Whole Cannabis vs Isolated CBD: Which Is Better?

If THC could induce psychosis in some people with mental disorders, is it better to just use pure CBD? The father from the United Patients Group reported his son had great results with cannabis strains that had a CBD:THC ratio of 20:1, but he also said they had even better results with isolated CBD in oil form. Another man claims that CBD oil was so effective he was able to quit his conventional antipsychotic prescription.

But the way that THC and CBD interact may also be important. In 2012, a man named Miles Houser wrote to a Harvard professorwho was collecting case studies on cannabis, stating that after running the gamut of conventional anticonvulsants, antipsychotics, and antidepressants, high-CBD cannabis had been the only thing that worked for him. In an article for the online magazine Ladybud, marijuana legalization advocate Gradi Jordan wrote that, based on the 36 years she'd used cannabis to treat her bipolar disorder, she felt THC was an essential component to effectively managing severe symptoms.

What's the bottom line? We still don't know. There's a lot of evidence that CBD—either in isolated form or in high-CBD strains of cannabis—can effectively treat both the manic and depressive symptoms of bipolar disorder. But most clinical cannabis studies don't include the ratio of CBD:THC in the strands they use, and more research is needed to explore whether CBD oil or whole cannabis works better. Like any psychedelic, cannabis needs to be treated with caution and respect, and it shouldn't be used as a haphazard self-medication. And as with all medicines, treatment is ultimately a matter of personal preference: the effectiveness and side effects will depend on the unique biochemistry and personality of each person. But while we're waiting on conclusive research, it seems that CBD is providing promising relief to people who need it.

Cannabis Use in Bipolar Disorder Presents a Treatment Challenge

**Abigail Nover**

Among patients with bipolar disorder, cannabis is the most commonly abused drug. Lifetime use of cannabis among bipolar patients is estimated to be around 70%, and 30% present a comorbidity of cannabis abuse or dependence. The risk for psychotic disorders increases with the frequency and intensity of cannabis use. Researchers have found that cannabis use is also associated with a younger age at onset of first manic episode, increased manic and depressive episodes, increased risk of rapid cycling, poorer outcome, and poorer treatment compliance.[1]

These findings illuminate the challenges in treating patients with bipolar disorder who use cannabis, especially as an increasing number of US states legalize marijuana. Self-medication with cannabis was recently found to be 3.73 percentage points higher among those living in states with medical marijuana laws.2Although further investigations are needed to clarify the relationship between mania onset and cannabis use, researchers say they are "undeniably correlated."1

Psychiatry Advisor spoke with Girish Subramanyan, MD, a psychiatrist in full-time private practice in San Francisco, California, specializing in the treatment of adults with mood and anxiety disorders, including treatment-resistant mood and anxiety disorders.

Psychiatry Advisor: Does cannabis use present any challenges in treating patients with bipolar disorder? If so, what are the challenges and how do they affect treatment?

**Dr Girish Subramanyan**: Yes. It can complicate the management of bipolar disorder by virtue of causing mood instability and psychosis in certain patients with bipolar disorder. Cannabis is a known psychotogenic drug for some people, although the majority of people who use it do not develop psychosis. But, among those that do, there seems to be a higher risk for conversion to schizophrenia and bipolar disorders, unfortunately. Moreover, it's not uncommon for me to see patients with bipolar disorder relapse into mania with recent cannabis use. Observational studies have demonstrated a correlation between cannabis use and hypomanic and manic relapse in bipolar disorder.

**Psychiatry Advisor**: Are there distinct challenges or effects of cannabis use in patients with bipolar I vs bipolar II?

**Dr Subramanyan**: Yes. The possibility of cannabis contributing to manic relapse in bipolar I disorder makes it potentially more dangerous in bipolar I disorders. Manias have the potential to cause devastating consequences in the lives of patients and their families. Plus, there is a real possibility that cannabis can contribute to psychotic manic episodes. This risk is probably lower in individuals with bipolar II disorder, but it is possible, I suppose, that someone with a true diagnosis of bipolar II disorder could have a cannabis-induced manic episode with psychotic features, something that may never have occurred spontaneously for this individual.

In bipolar II disorder, you may end up seeing more mood instability, mixed states, and hypomanic episodes, and although these states are uncomfortable, and even dangerous, if they are accompanied by suicidal ideations, they generally don't do as much damage as full-blown manic episodes.

**Psychiatry Advisor**: Has the legalization of recreational marijuana use in California had any noticeable effect on your treatment of bipolar disorder?

**Dr Subramanyan**: Surprisingly, I don't think I've seen much in the way of increased incidence of mania or psychosis in my practice since the legalization of recreational marijuana in California. What I have noticed, however, is that more and more patients in my practice are using some kind of cannabinoid for a variety of reasons: treatment of anxiety, treatment of pain, treatment of insomnia, etc. Patients seem to be using cannabidiol (CBD) products, in particular, more frequently. CBD is interesting in that it seems to have opposite effects in the brain as does THC.

There is a thought that it could actually have antipsychotic function.

**Amanda Hasten:** I was diagnosed with dipolar disorder at age 12. I always knew I was different because, one minute I'd be happy, [the] next minute I was crying, and then it all became too much and I ended up trying to commit suicide at 14. I was prescribed all kinds of medication, but nothing seemed to work. At the age of 16 years, I began smoking marijuana and my life was changed. No longer do I have these constant mood changes, and my mind doesn't run a mile a minute with dread and fear. I have a medical marijuana card now as an adult, and I am grateful to the marijuana industry for saving my life.

Nicholas G.: I have been struggling with and managing my manic and depressive episodes since 2004. I experience a lesser form of mania called hypomania, which means that although I may not experience grandiosity or psychosis like those with a bipolar 1 diagnosis, my behaviors are impulsive and have lasting consequences. This has cost me educational and professional opportunities, relationships, and even a bankruptcy. When I am on my prescribed meds I am able to reduce the frequency and severity of my manic and depressive episodes, but they will never completely go away.

I began using cannabis as a senior in high school. I increased my cannabis use as an undergrad when, unbeknownst to me, I began using cannabis to self-medicate. I had never seen a psychiatrist and knew little about mental health, but I did notice that smoking indica-heavy cannabis helped me sleep better and was one of the only methods I had ever discovered that slows my manic thoughts to a manageable level (which is why I stay far away from anything sativa, as that accelerates my thinking and makes things much worse). I used cannabis to stimulate my appetite when depression and anxiety made it too difficult to eat, and as a common activity with friends to help maintain a supportive network of friends. I stopped using cannabis completely for 6 years after I was initially diagnosed and stabilized on psychotropic medication. Unfortunately, once...I lost my insurance and was no longer able to afford to see my psychiatrist or pay for my medications...I turned back to cannabis to help manage my symptoms. The psychotropic medications are essential for me to maintain stable mental [health], but cannabis helps make things a little softer and more manageable.

www.ingramcontent.com/pod-product-compliance
Lightning Source LLC
Chambersburg PA
CBHW070515220526
45467CB00002B/672